Revealed: Aging In Superb Confidence

New Amazing Approach to preparing for an Enjoyable Old Age

By Lisa D. Douglas

All rights reserved. No part of this publication may be reproduced, distributed, or transmitted in any form or by any means, including photocopying, recording, or other electronic or mechanical methods, without the prior written permission of the publisher, except in the case of brief quotations embodied in critical reviews and certain other noncommercial uses permitted by copyright law.

Copyright © Lisa D. Douglas, 2022.

Table of Contents

Chapter 1

Determine how you want to look at old age

At one's youthful years it's of utmost importance to critically think through how healthy you would want to be at old age. We all mostly look at old people with a feeling of worry and sadness in our hearts towards them because obviously at old age your spouse might have passed on and your children might have left your house to pursue their own dreams leaving you all alone. This loneliness if not managed well can lead to your early demise. Hence the importance to acknowledge all these at a younger age and conscientise yourself on how you will handle yourself when these realities set in because it's all going to affect your health.

Some people use all their lifetime investment on hospital bills and drugs just to keep on living. You don't want this to be you, start now to invest in your health and make it a part of you so you will still be looking like forty years when you hit your sixties.

As we grow older, we experience an increasing number of major life changes, including career transitions and retirement, children leaving home, the loss of loved ones, physical and health challenges—and even a loss of independence. How we handle and grow from these changes is often the key to healthy aging.

Coping with change is difficult at any age and it's natural to feel the losses you experience. However, by balancing your sense of loss with positive factors, you can stay healthy and continue to reinvent yourself as you pass through landmark ages of 60, 70, 80, and beyond.

As well as learning to adapt to change, healthy aging also means finding new things you enjoy, staying physically and socially active, and feeling connected to your community and loved ones. Unfortunately, for many of us aging also brings anxiety and fear. How will I take care of myself late in life? What if I lose my spouse? What is going to happen to my mind?

Many of these fears stem from popular misconceptions about aging. But the truth is that you are stronger and more resilient than you may realize.

Staying healthy is important at any age, but for seniors, it is even more important for living a long, happy and active life.

Determining how healthy you want to be early in one's lifetime will enable you to take the right steps, be it your choice of occupation or financial investment decisions as you age so you can live a stress free life at old age.

Continue to maintain a healthy lifestyle and make adjustments for any changes in your function (e.g., hearing, vision, flexibility or strength).

Continue to engage in routine preventive health behaviors (e.g., get immunizations for flu and pneumonia).

Advocate for yourself and your family in health care settings or bring a knowledgeable representative with you. Do not be afraid to ask questions or get a second opinion.

If you feel anxious, depressed or are using alcohol or drugs to manage your mood, seek assistance . Untreated mental health problems are associated with poor physical health outcomes, including increased disability and illness as well as decreased quality of life
Be an interested person. Remain aware of new developments in the arts, sciences, politics and other areas of cultural and social interest.
Be an interesting person. Engage in something that matters to you and that you care passionately about.

Chapter 2

Make achievable/realistic goals

As we have different personalities and genes, we can not all aspire to achieve a common health goal. It is of utmost importance to know yourself and which healthy choices to make.
This is where adequate medical attention is so much needed so that you can have timely medical advice tailored to your specific need.

Make realistic goals. Example don't indulge in jumping rope each morning when you've been advised medically to only walk for 30 minutes daily because when it comes to health matters there are no second chances.
You've heard it time and again: physical activity and exercise are good for you, and you should aim to

make them part of your routine. There are countless studies that prove the important health benefits associated with exercise, and it becomes more important as we age. Regular physical activity and exercise for seniors helps improve mental and physical health, both of which will help you maintain your independence as you age.
You take the wrong exercise for example and it might bring adverse consequences.

As you get older, it can be easy to find excuses to let yourself slow down. However, exercise is vitally important for aging. Exercise improves your quality of life, meaning everything from how much activity we can do, to what kind of mood we're in.
Little efforts are better than no efforts at all. Just do what you ve been

advised medically to do and be committed to it.

Chapter 3

Have a sound financial state

Having a sound financial state at old age is so important. Many aged people are stuck at home with even some of them begging constantly to feed and care for themselves.
Please this point is so key because financial stress at old age must be totally eradicated if you want to enjoy your old age.

The mistake most people make, especially Africans, is overly dependent on their children and relatives at old age forging that their children and relatives also have their own lives to live. Once reality sets in and these children are unable to meet their expectations, then they become disappointed and are left at the mercy of nature to decide what happens to them.

We all give so much to support our children to have great futures but if you are not careful you might think they owe you a pay back at your old age which is highly risky. If you're blessed to have your children acknowledge your immense support in their lives and wants to appreciate you financially at old your old age, it's should just be a bonus but don't let it be your sole reliance because you may be disappointed and that will definitely be a huge stress on you which can lead to your early demise.

The years between 65 and 80 are often referred to as the "golden years," a time when older adults have retired, are likely living without dependents, and yet still have the physical and cognitive ability to do as they please. However, the golden years—and the years that follow—lose their luster if and when an older adult does not have the finances to live comfortably, let alone retire.

Financial independence is a critical aspect of older adulthood, yet it is not a factor that is always considered or prepared for properly. Many find themselves facing unexpected costs that can't be afforded and/or without the resources to continue living where and how they want.

It would greatly benefit older adults, and in fact adults of all ages, to better understand the complexities of financial independence as a senior citizen, as well as the barriers that exist in attaining such stability. Equally, those who serve young, middle-aged, and older adults, such as social workers, would be better able to provide useful services by also building their knowledge base.

Although they're not financial managers, social workers can and do assist clients in working toward and maintaining financial independence through older adulthood.

Many of the benefits of getting your financial house in order are obvious. But there are some lesser-known reasons to get it together in the money department you may have overlooked...

Less stress and better health. In a survey conducted by the American Psychological Association, 73% of people listed money as the number one factor affecting their stress level. This is a problem because persistent stress isn't just unpleasant—it's deadly. Stress is a significant contributor to a host of serious physical ailments like heart disease, stroke, depression, and even obesity. By doing the work necessary to get your financial house in order, you might also add some years, and greater quality, to your life.

Better marriages. Money woes are hard on relationships. The inevitable day of reckoning (like when the credit card bill is due, or the mortgage is in foreclosure) can bring out the finger-pointing and cause couples to turn on one another, rather than work together to fix the problem. Couples with a sound, mutually-negotiated financial plan may not get everything they want, but they're less likely to blame one another for it.

More options in life. When you manage money well and plan for tomorrow, you have greater control over your own life. Those who are constantly mired in heavy debt, by contrast, are slaves to their payments and what the banks will allow them to do. Want to have the financial margin needed to make a career change? Want to have more choices related to your kids' education? Then make small sacrifices now that will empower you later.

The freedom to be generous. People who are financially stable have more margin. In other words, they don't live to the end (or beyond) of their means. They build in a bit of a buffer in the financial plan for the "what ifs" in life. That's a wonderful feeling when you're suddenly confronted with a need or a cause that you desperately want to support...and you have the means to do so.

More financially stable kids. Kids who grow up in a family culture of financial literacy and accountability have a greater chance of being financially stable in their own adult lives. And trust us, it's a wonderful thing to have adult children who can take care of themselves and don't need to revisit the parental well over and over in adulthood to make ends meet. But don't assume they'll learn it all by osmosis. Be intentional in teaching the basics of money management to your kids.

When you're still in your 50s, it's wise to have a life insurance plan in place. There are several options for those over 50; keep in mind that insurance policy premiums increase as you age. There are several advantages in taking out a policy in your 50s. First, you probably will not need a medical examination to sign up for one. Second, you will have a fixed premium that will not change, among other advantages. The bulk that will be received from the insurance can save your loved ones from a lot of financial troubles after you're gone.

Rather than entrusting your old age to your children or relatives, take charge and be solely responsible of your own old age and ensure to save much and put financial structures in place to continue to support you throughout old age and leave a good legacy behind

Chapter 4

Do your best to raise your children Right while being consciously concerned with your extended family

Teach a child the way he should go and as he grows he shall not depart from it, says the Good book .People often use this verse as a guarantee that if you raise your children "in the discipline and instruction of God,they'll always stay on the right path. That interpretation can be problematic, particularly for the "good parents" I know who have seen their older children stray from the faith. We all know that we can try our best, and sometimes the results are different than we would have hoped.

God has given us free will to make our own choices, after all.

This is not a promise to parents who raise their children properly but a warning to those who allow their adolescents to grow up without guidance, who raise them to go their own way." Children left to their own way are not likely to change; they'll become adults who go their own way... the wrong way.Folly as the Good book tells us is bound up in the heart of a child which means obviously l that children don't tend to make wise choices on their own.

It's about parents helping their children discover their purpose and path in life. Parents are in the unique role of helping children discover how God has equipped them and how they can use their gifts in a positive way as adults.

You have a responsibility as parents to teach our children what matters in life as they have been entrusted into your care.

Our children are going to learn about the world around them and their role in it. If they don't learn from us, they will learn from someone else. It's our responsibility to use our time with our kids wisely.

You have influence as a parent.

Children are sponges. And, they seem to soak up everything – good and bad. I'm supposed to live and love. Also children are in your care and looking for your example children often imitate us. They learn how to act by seeing how we act. They'll only know how to love by seeing how we love.I've often thought about it this way: the moon reflects light from the sun. It's not a big mirror in the sky reflecting the sun exactly, or else the light from the moon and sun would be the same. When the moon is full, it looks quite bright. But, even at its brightest, it reflects less than 20 percent of the sun's light. That was the intention... for the moon to be the "lesser light."

What you do as a parent matters and it will lead to results. Our children are going to become adults, whether we want them to grow up or not!
The years our children are in our homes are critical. These are the formative years when they are developing their entire worldview.

Your inability to raise your children well is obviously going to be a big burden on you at your old age because they will always bring you problems which you can not ignore.

This will surely bring you constant stress which will be a big toll on your total health.

You don't want any of these, it will be such a great gain to try all you can to train and raise these children properly to guarantee your peace of mind and awesome health when you age.

It's also imperative to have a close and perfect relationship with your extended family and support them whether financially or any way you can. It's not advisable to live in isolation when aging. Your extended family will be of great support and will give you a great sense of belonging as you have the opportunity to spend time with your loved ones. Elderly people might feel lonely when they do not have their closed ones around them but living closely with their family members can make you feel happy.

Chapter 5

Regular medical check ups

Studies show that about 10% fewer adults have annual contact with a medical professional when compared to kids. Although this may not be surprising, wellness visits are extremely important.

Today's wellness exams go beyond the standard physical, allowing doctors to identify preventive measures that will keep you healthier and save you money.
While exercise, a balanced diet, and a healthy lifestyle are important to keep oneself healthy, it is also very important to go for health checkups at periodic intervals.
Why do you need to go for a Regular Medical Checkup?

Going for a medical checkup regularly helps you avoid a wide number of diseases and catch other diseases early on. It also serves to keep you better-advised about your health, keep your physician or other doctors apprised on your health, and basically result in a healthier life.

1. Going for a Medical Checkup regularly can reduce your risk of getting sick

Regular medical checkups include a number of physical and mental checks, making sure that your body and mind are fit and fine. These checkups are known as full body checkups for this reason – because they examine you from head to toe, almost literally.

The reason this is done is to catch any disease early on, and so that you can be prescribed the right treatment for it.

2. Regular Checkups can help identify stress-related diseases
These days with factors such as the heavy Kathmandu traffic, constant pressure at work (or school, college), unpredictable weather, it is no surprise that most people are suffering from stress.
This is causing higher levels of stress in everyone and may even result in stress-related diseases and disorders which can manifest physically or even psychologically.
A regular full body checkup will help your doctor diagnose such issues and also give you the opportunity to discuss stress to get the treatment that you need.

3. Yearly Checkups can help to identify blood test results

Most people know the symptoms of common diseases such as cold or a fever since these usually have physical symptoms. While this may suffice for smaller diseases, you may be suffering from something worse which can get worse without going for a checkup.

It is for this reason that doctors usually ask for a blood test, which is also an essential part of any yearly health checkup package (although the exact tests can differ depending on your age and lifestyle).

These blood tests further help screen out various potential diseases.

4. Periodic Health Checkups will make you more aware of your health

Many people take their health for granted, and most of us rarely visit a hospital or a doctor until we are actually sick and need treatment. This also makes us more likely to make poorer decisions regarding our health, especially when it comes to exercise and the food we eat.

Going for a period health checkup automatically will make you more aware of your health and what you can to lead a healthier lifestyle. This is partly because of just the act of visiting the hospital and speaking to your doctor, as well as seeing other patients and hospital visitors.

5. Yearly Full Body Checkups can reduce healthcare costs over time
As mentioned earlier, going for Full Body Checkups and other types of preventive checkups regularly helps prevent, and avoid diseases as well as treat other diseases at an early stage.

This in turn reduces the chance of you getting sick (or more sick) which further reduces your medical costs.

Let's also not forget the time factor – getting sick can result in needing to take time off from work or school and can disrupt your entire lifestyle.

A medical checkup every now and then ensures that you are healthy and decreases the chances of having to take a sick day, or even get admitted to the hospital.

What kind of Health Checkup Package should I choose?

Most hospitals and health providers will have a number of Preventive Health Checkup Packages available. These differ by the tests involved based on your age and lifestyle.

E.g. younger people may need fewer screening since they are relatively more healthy. Older people will probably need a health package that includes cardiac screening tests since they are more at risk.

Chapter 6

Eating Right

As you get older, eating well can help improve your mental sharpness, boost your energy levels, and increase your resistance to illness.

The benefits of healthy eating as you age
Healthy eating is important at any age, but becomes even more so as we reach midlife and beyond. As well as keeping your body healthy, eating well can also be the key to a positive outlook and staying emotionally balanced. But healthy eating doesn't have to be about dieting and sacrifice. Rather, it should be all about enjoying fresh, tasty food, wholesome ingredients, and eating in the company of friends and family.

No matter your age or your previous eating habits, it's never too late to change your diet and improve the way you think and feel. Improving your diet now can help you to:

Live longer and stronger. Good nutrition can boost immunity, fight illness-causing toxins, keep weight in check, and reduce the risk of heart disease, stroke, high blood pressure, cancer etc.

Along with physical activity, a balanced diet can also contribute to enhanced independence as you age.

Sharpen your mind. People who eat fruit, leafy veggies, and fish and nuts packed with omega-3 fatty acids may be able to improve focus and decrease their risk of Alzheimer's disease. Antioxidant-rich green tea may also enhance memory and mental alertness as you age.

Feel better. Wholesome meals can give you more energy and help you look better, resulting in a boost to your mood and self-esteem. It's all connected—when your body feels good, you feel happier inside and out. Healthy eating is about more than just food

Eating well as you age is about more than just the quality and variety of your food. It's also about the pleasure of eating, which increases when a meal is shared. Eating with others can be as important as adding vitamins to your diet. A social atmosphere stimulates your mind, makes meals more enjoyable, and can help you stick to your healthy eating plan.

Even if you live alone, you can make healthy meals more pleasurable by:
Shopping with others. Shopping with a friend can give you a chance to

catch up without falling behind on your chores. It's also a great way to share new meal ideas and save money on discount deals like "buy one, get the second half price".

Cooking with others. Invite a friend to share cooking responsibilities—one prepares the entrée, the other dessert, for example. Cooking with others can be a fun way to deepen your relationships, and splitting costs can make it cheaper for both of you.

Making mealtimes a social experience. The simple act of talking to a friend or loved over the dinner table can play a big role in relieving stress and boosting mood. Gather the family together regularly and stay up to date on everyone's lives. Invite a friend, coworker, or neighbor over.

As you get older, your nutritional needs, appetite, and food habits can change in several ways.

Calories:

You'll probably need fewer calories as you age to maintain a healthy weight. Eating more calories than you burn leads to weight gain.

You may find you have less energy and more muscle or joint problems as you get older. As a result, you may become less mobile and burn fewer calories through physical activity. You may also lose muscle mass. This causes your metabolism to slow down, lowering your caloric needs.

Appetite:

Many people experience a loss of appetite with age. It's also common for your sense of taste and smell to diminish. This can lead you to eat less.

If you're burning fewer calories through physical activity, eating less may not be a problem. However, you need to get enough calories and nutrients to maintain healthy organs, muscles, and bones. Not getting enough can lead to malnutrition and health problems.

Medical Conditions:

As you age, you become more susceptible to chronic health problems, such as diabetes, high blood pressure, high cholesterol, and osteoporosis. To help prevent or treat these conditions, your doctor may recommend changes to your diet.

For example, if you've been diagnosed with diabetes, high blood pressure, or high cholesterol, you should eat foods that are rich in nutrients, but low in excess calories, processed sugars, and saturated and trans fats. Your doctor may also advise you to eat less sodium.

Some older adults become sensitive to foods such as onions, peppers, dairy products, and spicy foods. You may need to cut some of these foods out of your diet.

Medications:
You may need to take medications to manage chronic health conditions. Some medications can affect your appetite. Some can also interact with certain foods and nutritional supplements.
If you're taking medication, be sure to check with your doctor or pharmacist to find out whether you need to make any changes to your diet.

Oral Health:
Old people have their own set of oral health concerns. Some of these can interfere with your ability to eat. For example, dentures that don't fit

properly may lead to poor eating habits and malnutrition. Infections in your mouth can also cause problems.

Immune System:
Your immune system weakens with age. This raises your risk of food-borne illness, or food poisoning. Proper food safety techniques are important at every age. However, you may need to take extra precautions as your immune system weakens.

Home Life:
Losing a spouse or other family members can impact your daily habits, including your eating patterns. You may feel depressed, which can lead to lower appetite. If your family member did most of the cooking, you might not know how to prepare food for yourself. Some people simply choose not to eat,

rather than cook a meal for themselves.

If you're finding it difficult to prepare food for yourself, talk to a family member, trusted friend, or your doctor. Depending on your area, there may be services available to help make sure you're getting the food you need.

Chapter 7

Good sleep

A good night's sleep is essential for successful aging, no matter how old you are. After all, sleep is a time of rest and rejuvenation, when our minds and bodies can recuperate after a long day. We spend about 1/3 of our lives sleeping, and quality sleep is a vital indicator of overall health and well-being], especially for older adults.

Usually people over age 65 should get at least seven-to-eight hours of sleep every night. That's because getting the rest you need can help you stay both physically and mentally well as you age.

A good night's sleep boosts your mood.

Sleep and mental health are closely related. In many ways, both impact each other. Not getting enough sleep can lead to mental health issues like depression and anxiety, while mental health conditions can, in turn, lower your sleep quality. A good night's sleep is crucial for your mental well-being.

Quality sleep lowers your risk of diseases.

Lack of sleep increases your risk of serious health conditions like high blood pressure, cardiovascular disease, diabetes and obesity. Studies show that insufficient sleep puts added stress on the body, leading to inflammation and a weakened immune system. During sleep, our bodies undergo restorative functions like muscle growth, protein synthesis and tissue repair – all of which are needed to keep your immune system strong.

Restful sleep maintains your weight and supports metabolism.
Getting enough sleep is key to weight maintenance and keeping your metabolism moving at a healthy rate. Sufficient sleep also regulates ghrelin, a hormone that stimulates your appetite. If you're sleep deprived, your metabolism slows down which can lead to weight gain.

Good sleep improves concentration and memory.
A good night's rest keeps your brain healthy and your memory sharp. It's well known that sleep deprivation has a negative impact on your attention span and short-term memory. Lack of

sleep also weakens your decision-making ability and your long-term memory as well. And over time, too little sleep can even contribute to cognitive decline, memory loss and increase your risk for developing dementia.

Bedtime is when your brain clears harmful toxins.
Contrary to popular belief, our brains don't slow down while we're sleeping. Scientists are learning more about the glymphatic system, which serves as a waste disposal system in our bodies and clears harmful toxins and debris from our brains. The glymphatic system is almost 10 times more active during sleep than it is during wakefulness.

There's no "right" amount of sleep. What you consider a good amount can be entirely different than what your neighbor needs.

If you get fewer Zzz's than you did when you were younger, but you still feel rested and energetic, you might simply need less sleep than you used to.

What Can Cause Sleep Problems?

If you figure out what's keeping you up at night, you can tackle the issue and sleep better.

Illnesses and conditions. You may have a medical condition that's affecting your rest. Ailments like arthritis, sleep apnea, and restless legs syndrome can all make sleep a challenge. Treatment to help your condition may help you get some shut-eye.

Medications. Some can keep you awake at night. Make sure your doctor knows about all the medications you take. They may suggest you adjust when to take it or how much you take. They may even be able to change your medication to something that won't affect your slumber.

Change. The older you get, the more likely you are to have some major transitions in your life. Things like illness, financial problems, or the death of a loved one cause stress, and that can make it hard to sleep. Talk to your family or meet with a counselor to find ways to manage your stress.

Retirement. You might have a lot more downtime and be less active during the day. That can throw off your sleep-wake schedule. So try to keep your body and mind moving: You could volunteer, hit the gym, learn a new skill, spend time with friends and family -- the point is, stay active.

We can never underestimate the Importance of sleep in our lives, especially as you age. Have time to sleep properly to boost your health and look fresher and stronger than your peers as you age.

Chapter 8

Moderate social life

Socialization is even recommended for pets! Socialization is the activity of mixing socially with others. It's intended to foster relationships, establish good communication skills, and promote a sense of community. Maintaining strong social ties is important for aging adults to feel a sense of purpose and avoid feelings of loneliness or depression.I

People who perceive their friends and family members as supportive during times of need have a stronger sense of meaning in their lives; that is, they live their lives with a broader purpose, adhering to a value system that fits within the larger social world.

The importance of socialization never wears off, and it's particularly relevant at old age. Here's why.
Socializing keeps people young at heart, emotionally vibrant, and mentally sharp. As you, you age, have you taken time to consider the continued importance of socialization? When you were a baby, socialization helped you develop who you are. As you are aging,it remains important that you have a social life to help maintain a healthy physical and emotional balance.

Socializing can provide a number of benefits to your physical and mental health. Did you know that connecting with friends may also boost your brain health and lower your risk of diseases? If you need reasons to help justify spending extra time lingering

over coffee or a puzzle, memory loss was identified as a key measuring stick in older adults. There is evidence that suggests memory loss is a strong risk factor for dementia, which currently impacts a great deal for people over the age of 65.
Social isolation is one of the leading causes of depression in older people.

Loneliness can easily take its toll on individuals of every age, but there's greater concern for older adults as routines and independence changes. Socialization can have a positive effect where isolation is concerned by helping the aged feel loved and needed.
Lives can be affirmed by the activities and interactions. Being around other people, especially spending time doing something fun or rewarding, helps individuals keep a positive

outlook on life and a healthy mental state.

Older adults with active social lives can also prevent a number of physical ailments from negatively impacting their overall health. When you maintain an active physical regimen with friends and neighbors, you reap the reward in terms of improved physical health as you age. Adults of all ages are encouraged to remain physically active, significantly boosting their overall health as they age.

More importantly, older people who remain physically and intellectually active in social settings can also help fight off depression through interaction.

Chapter 9

Conclusion

How will it feel like to live life from birth through teens to youthful years to adulthood only to have unrest and no peace of mind at old age when actually that is the time you need it the MOST.

Thus it behooves you as you are not there yet to think through what you really want your old age to be like and carefully put measures and structures in place to enable you to have a great and awesome old age.

Getting ready for old age needs a plan. Starting a plan too late in life will overwhelm you and make you feel like you are running a marathon. Not only will you be able to live comfortably while planning for your future, but you will also enjoy your life even more when you retire. You can spend every year after adopting a healthy lifestyle to feel safe and secure, and to have more time to do all the things you might have missed out on before.

With these preparations in place, you will definitely be looking like age 40 when you actually clock age 70.

www.ingramcontent.com/pod-product-compliance
Lightning Source LLC
Chambersburg PA
CBHW072050150726
47996CB00015B/2467